ISBN 978-1-234-56789-1

Contents

Introduction

Hello, I'm Saffron Baldoza. I'm 14 years old and I organised this anthology in aid of B-eat. B-eat is a charity dedicated to helping young people with eating disorders.

I was introduced to B-eat through my Citizenship GCSE. We had to become a support group for a charity – and so my group chose B-eat. The 4 other members of my talented group have helped me in creating this book, from sharing informative research to encouraging other people to contribute to the book.

One of our aims as a support group for B-eat was to raise awareness of the charity and how serious eating disorders are. It was at that point that I thought of the idea of creating an anthology of people's work to self-publish and sell; with all the profits going to B-eat.

It was then decided that I would organise this book. This was mainly because I have become the most passionate for supporting this charity. When I was 9 I was diagnosed with Anorexia Nervosa. It has been a long struggle for me, and I have always used art and writing as creative therapy for me. At 14, my peers and I are at a common age to not only suffer from eating disorders but to feel especially pressured from schoolwork and criticism. My age group are more susceptible to worrying about our appearances, and so I imagined people's contributions to the book would be both thought-provoking and appropriate.

This book contains the work of a small handful of talented individuals who kindly have shared their creativity with only a thank you in return. I would like to personally thank them for making this book possible. Not many people gave up their time for this project, however we received enough contributions to produce it.

This book contains not only poems but various writing pieces, as well as some pieces of photography and art. You will see that a few of the projects have an unnamed author; this was a decision made only by the author for their own privacy. Others also have just the first name of the author written – this was again because of their own personal wishes.

Thank you for purchasing and reading this book. We appreciate your interest in our work, and for supporting B-eat,

Saffron Baldoza

POETRY

Reflections

Stop.
Pause.

Your face crumples like a house of cards
Glimmering tear-tracks
Sparkling like morning dew.
Your breath catches
Lodged in your throat
Lodged in your heart:
An illness you cannot break.
Pinching hollows beneath your cheeks
Sunken eyes searching frantically
For every flaw.

Ugly UglyUgly
You will never look like
That girl in the magazine:
Perfect, pretty, posed,
That girl at the bus stop:
Flawless, effortless,
That friend:
The definition of perfect.

Fat FatFat.
Maybe if you starve
Until you wear your bones
Like a fashion statement –
"This is who I am"

Maybe if you shred your skin
Until it hangs like crimson ribbons
Drenched with blood-stained sorrow.
Maybe if you slice open your heart
And bury it in society's little box of treasures.
Maybe.

Not skinny.
Not skinny.
Not skinny.

Anonymous

Cover Girl

She is the perfect image
of emaciated cool
and nicely starved.
She is just 8 inches
of low-fat, no-sugar ink
and airbrushed thighs.

And yet her body
is dyed onto each ripple
of your brain.
And her figure has been stretched
over what is left
Of you.

Her image has been distorted;
fragility ruined by solidity and
new world feminity.
Her beauty has been
Purged on Disney princesses and
Society's drunken dreams.

She might be past
the idea of sexy curves
and womanly waists.
But she simply laughs at you,
your hollowed cheeks,
ringing truths.

Anonymous

<u>Worthy</u>

I look at you:
Perfection.
Intelligent, Funny, Kind –
I could never be worthy of you.
I gaze in the mirror:
Ugly magnified.
Something for the world to laugh and spit at –
Then leave to die.

But if my bones burst out of my
Paper thin skin
Then, will you talk to me?
And when my arms look like
Red velvet ribbons
Then, will you be friends with me?
And when my whole stomach
Screams with the pain
Then, will you try loving me?
And finally, when I'm lying
In a cheap coffin

Then, Will I be worthy of you?

Anonymous

Fairytale

She used to be happy;
She walked with her chin up high
She seemed to have self confidence
I would've believed she could fly.

But lately she's been looking down
Muttering numbers under her breath
Lost to the world of reality
It's like she's living dead.
But today she looked worse than usual
As if she was decaying, day by day
And Her hollowed cheeks glared at me
Despite the stuff she says
Tomorrow is the end for her
Or so the doctor said
She's done living with the illness
It's the illness that's been fed

She wasn't a fairytale princess
She set her dreams aside
She was cruelly tempted
And she never really tried.

Saffron Baldoza, 14

OTHER WRITING

Anorexia

Knowing someone with an eating disorder is hard, most especially when they are a close friend. You watch her crumbling on the inside as the feeling of helplessness overcomes your mind, dominating all other relatively trivial thoughts, pushing itself to the forefront of your mind each time you catch a glimpse of her withering mind and body. You panic again at how worn she looks.

It's eating her from the inside, as she continues to refuse to eat anything, sucking the life out of her. Your repeated offers of help are pushed aside as she bravely but rashly decides she needs to journey this road alone. Each day gets harder as the weeks draw by until she is left with almost nothing. All bridges broken, she slumps alone in her corner. Self-loathing overcomes as she wallows in her pain but a light draws her to her feet.

The burdens are gradually lifting as the world around her comes into focus again. An overwhelming sense of love washes over her. She has finally come to realize she is not alone and she can see an escape route from this barred cage. She is eating at last and she is binging but she doesn't care.

Her life is worth living again and the prospect of her bright future is now seriously considered rather than pushed aside and labelled 'impossible'. The sense of relief is unexplainable and seeing her now makes you smile. She was stronger than you could ever imagine and she has pulled through where others have fallen. I am just so glad she's so strong.

Becky, 13

The Truth

Everyday I'm forced to face the truth.

I look at myself; and all I want to do is cry. How could I let this happen? My friends don't look like this. How do they do it? No - How do they do it without being like me? I can feel every single one of my ribs, and the sharp curvatures of my hips jut out painfully, but it will never be enough when I can still see the fat. Spread over me. How come I can tell every pound I've put on, but never the ones I've taken off?

I feel the comforting points of my spine, slipping down from between the shoulder blades to my lower back – my eyes closed. If I close my eyes I can pretend it doesn't matter. I can kid myself that everything will be better if I just do what everyone says. That's how I get through the day:

Pretending.

Pretending if I just do what they say I'll get better. Pretending everything's going okay for me. Pretending that things are actually changing.

But all I can see is the fat. I've tried everything. Exercise in the mornings, cutting out the lunches. But I will never be able to look in the mirror and smile at my reflection. And then you wonder why there is nothing left for me to hold on to.

You wonder why I have scratched every day I hurt on my arm as a reminder. You wonder why I act like I have no hope when I still earnestly talk about the future like I truly believe in it.

Because that's all it really is, isn't it? Lack of belief.

But if I can see no way out of this, what is the point in still pretending? What is the point in throwing away my blades and instead keeping my lunches just to make people happy?

What's the point, when it's all for you? What's the point, when you could never ever love me?

What's the point, when I'll be in a coffin before you've read this?

What's the point?

Anonymous, 14

PHOTOGRAPHY AND ART

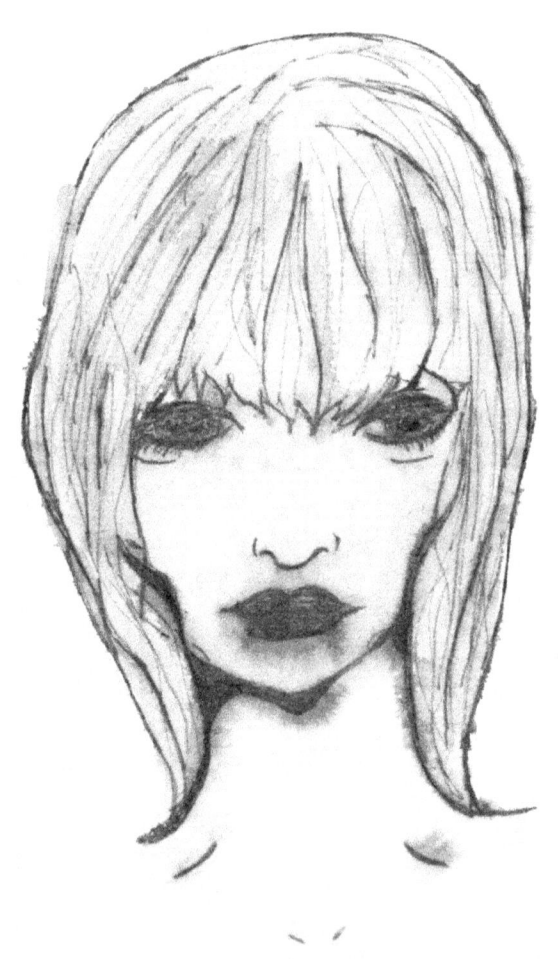

Helpless

I drew this girl to represent someone with the illness who knows their fate; they've gone too far and they know they won't ever be able to turn back. I read an article somewhere describing anorexia as a 'Slow Suicide'. Anorexia springs from a deep self hatred, and in this picture I tried to capture the regret of this girl, as well as the truth of the illness.

Saffron Baldoza, 14

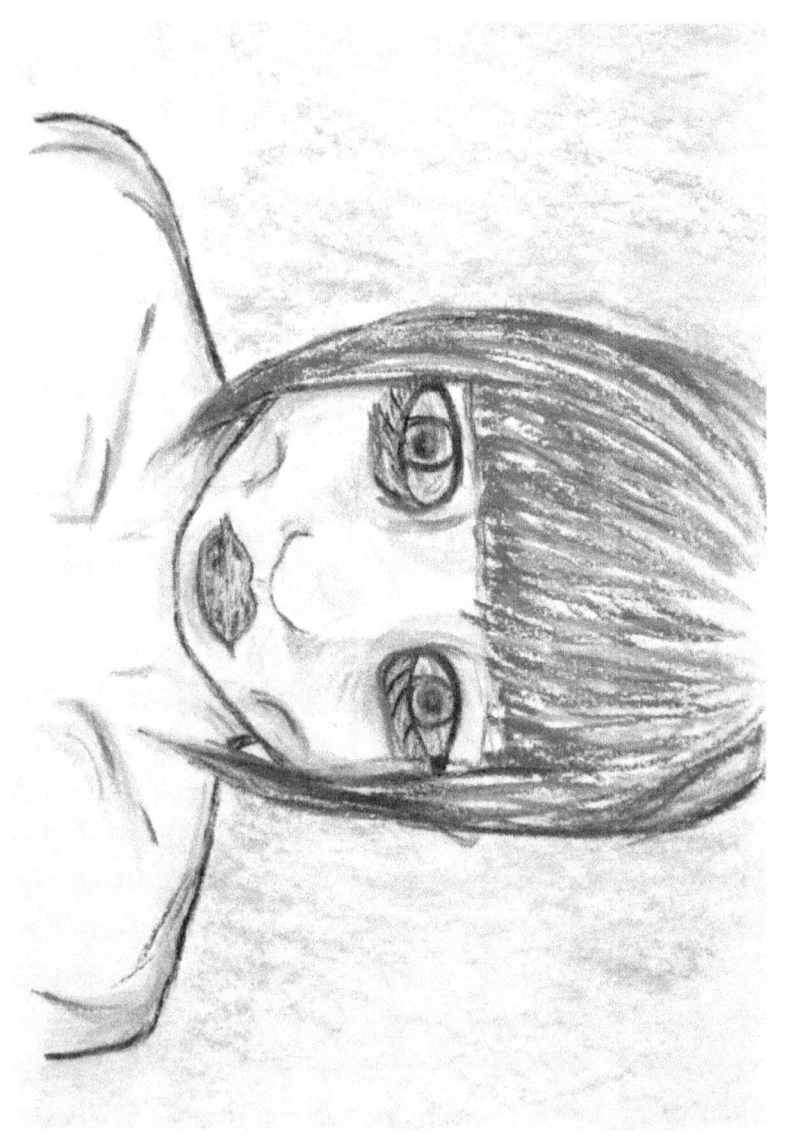

Landscape Picture

Controlled

I drew this girl to show how Anorexia takes over someone's life. The eyes of this girl are closed: but the eyes of the illness are wide open. They are the eyes that are always open and are all-seeing. These eyes will be her new eyes. They represent anorexia, which is controlling her.

Saffron Baldoza 14

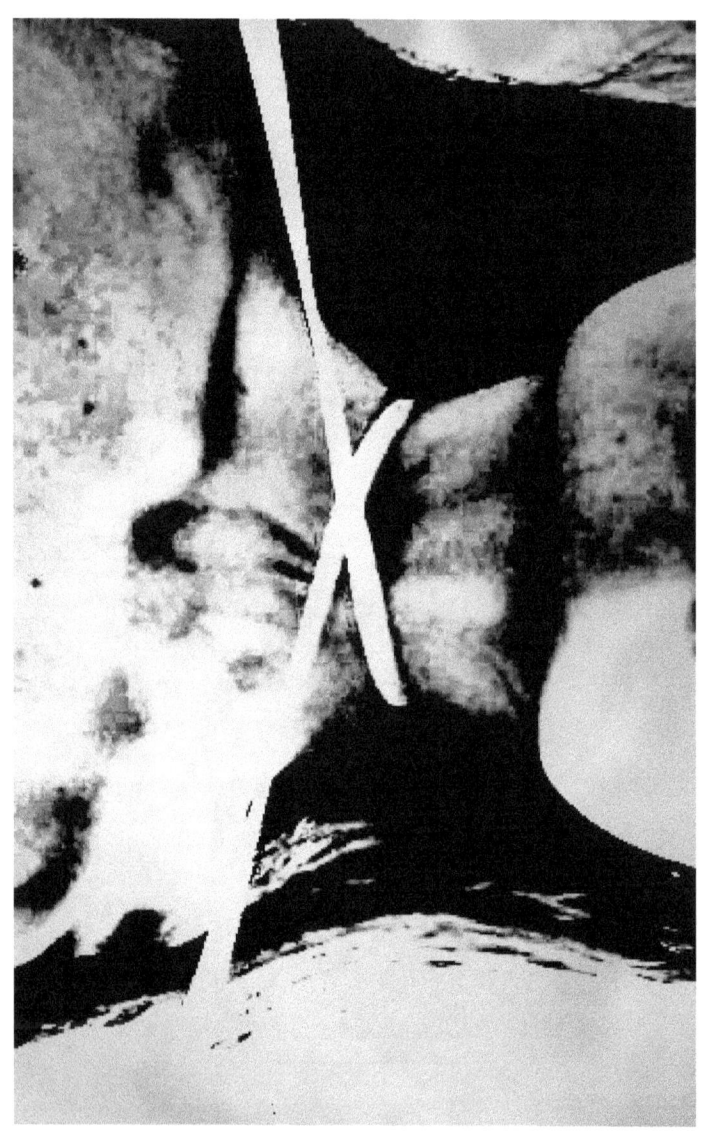

Landscape Photo

The Scaled Suicide

I took this photo because I wanted to shock people. Sometimes I think you need a slightly scary photo to jump out at people and shock them into realising how serious something is. The band round the girls neck could be anything, but is meant to be measuring tape. This photo shows how the numbers end up taking over a sufferer's life, and eventually driving them – quite often – near death.

Saffron Baldoza, 14

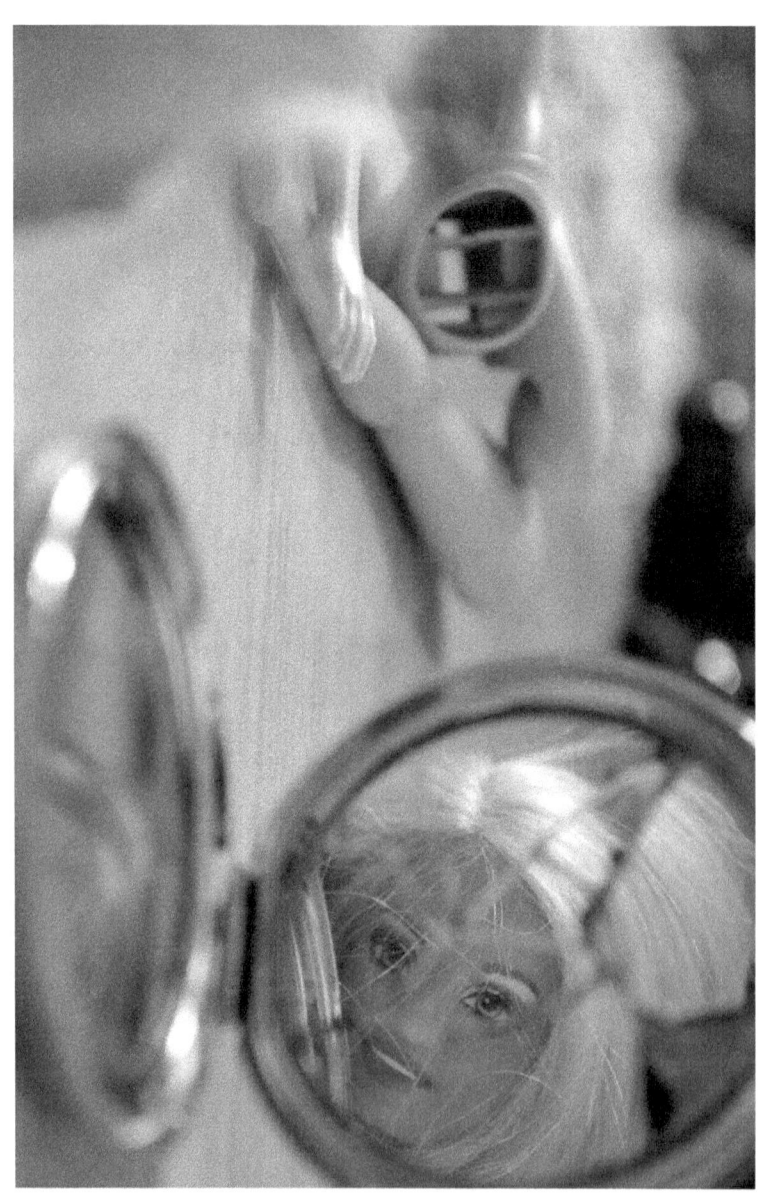

Landscape Photo

Seeking Barbie

I took this photo to emphasise what sufferers are looking for in the mirror. It isn't necessarily Barbie; but a lot of the time they are looking for perfection, or at least something that isn't there. This perfection or 'ideal' might be a friend, a model, an actress – or just a general want to be prettier.

I also wanted to show how out of proportion and unrealistic Barbie is – and how she could never be real. If Barbie was real, it is suggested she would have to walk on all fours. Additionally her BMI would be that which would be considered anorexic.

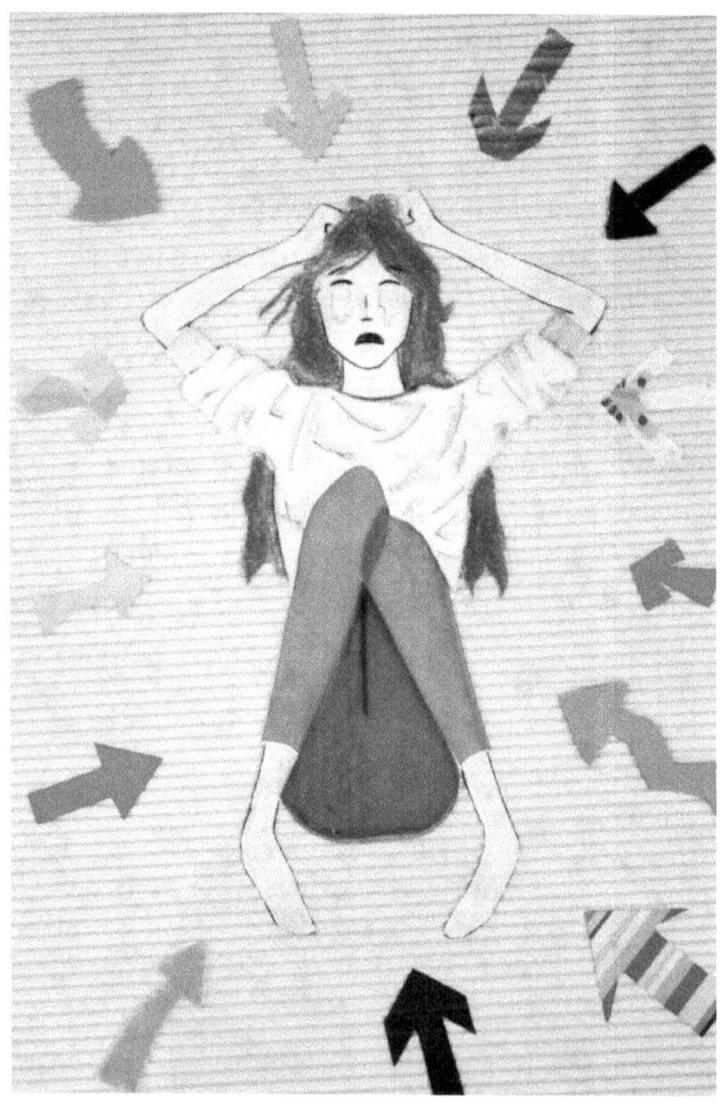

Anorexia

Florence Nicholls, 13

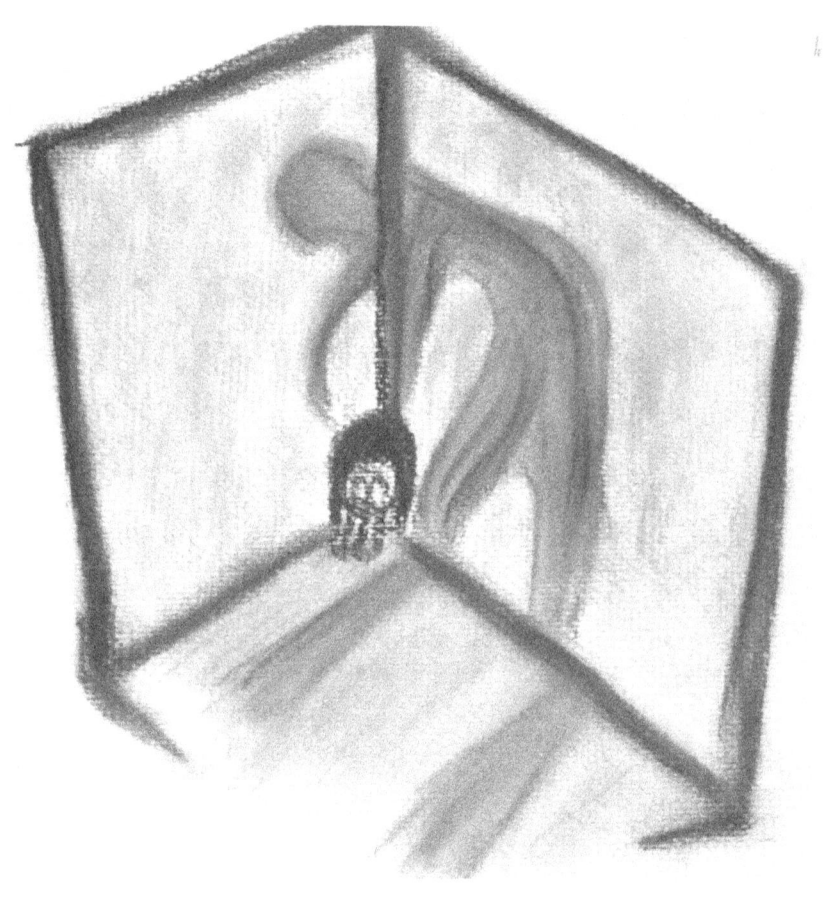

Vulnerability

Anonymous, 14

Ending Note

Thank you for taking the time to read through this book and seeing the work of a few 13/14 year olds. A lot of work and time has gone into this book: from creating the pieces to collecting them to organising them into it.

We hope this book will help to raise awareness of the charity and eating disorders, as well as give a unique insight to how young teenage girls visualise eating disorders and how eating disorders affect them. We are using the book to raise money for B-eat, but we want it to be informative and interesting too.

Below I'd like to thank everyone who didn't necessarily contribute a piece in the book but helped with creating it:

Nashrini Pather – *The other member of my group who took part in creating this book through advising me on the content as well as generals support.*

My Family – *Particularly my grandfather, who was very supporting in my big ambitions for this book and has been informative in how to organise and layout a book.*

Grace Bowman– Author of 'Thin', we contacted Grace Bowman and she kindly wrote back to us, sending us a video of her giving us information on eating disorders. Grace Bowman also gave us some advice and her best wishes on supporting B-eat.

Olivia Ray, Helena Meadows and Emily Dalton – The other three members of my Citizenship GCSE group.

PLEASE SUPPORT B-EAT AND HELP PEOPLE WITH EATING DISORDERS.

It is estimated that 10% of eating disorder sufferer's die as a result, but experts believe the number is actually much higher.

It is believed that only around 60% of anorexics recover in their lifetime.

Around 90% of all anorexic's are female.

Over a ¼ of anorexics are so weak that they require immediate hospitalisation.

The highest rates of anorexia are seen in female teenagers aged between 13 and 19.

50% of all girls between 13 and 15 think they are overweight.

40% of 9 year old girls have (attempted to) diet.

80% of 13 year old girls have (attempted to) diet.

Anorexia is the 3rd most common chronic illness in teenagers.